HOLISTIC HEALTH

FOR
PROPER GEEZERS
AND
CLASSY LADIES

by

Scott Bryant

"Get the body fitness you want"

Grosvenor House
Publishing Limited

The right of Scott Bryant to be identified as the author of this
work has been asserted in accordance with Section 78
of the Copyright, Designs and Patents Act 1988

This book is published by
Grosvenor House Publishing Ltd
Link House
140 The Broadway, Tolworth, Surrey, KT6 7HT.
www.grosvenorhousepublishing.co.uk

A CIP record for this book
is available from the British Library

ISBN 978-1-78623-466-7

"I highly recommend Scott, try and you will be satisfied!"

I had Scott as a personal trainer for many years, around 18 I can say that training with him is a part of my life. He helped me to stay young, to have a proper good posture, to remain flexible and to maintain a proper fit muscular body despite the age! I enjoy not only the physical training but also the discussion and advice on nutrition and wellness. He is very knowledgeable and I highly recommend Scott, try and you will be satisfied!

Dr Roberto Viel (plastic surgeon/author), **The London Centre for Aesthetic Surgery, Harley Street**

"More energy and more downtime, with less stress. Highly recommended".

Corrective Exercise has been gaining with Scott since January after fractured rib whilst skiing. As result I have completely renovated my diet, training program and lifestyle for the better, I am stronger, leaner and have more energy and more downtime, with less stress. Highly recommended.

Jane, **Physiotherapist, Harley Street**

"Scott trained me and the results have been extraordinary".

I've been working with Scott for 9 months with a real objective to improve my golf game. I have been aware of the Paul Chek approach to fitness and sports performance for some years, and with Scott training me the results have been extraordinary. We have worked on balance, strength, speed, and endurance and always with the mechanics of the golf swing as the key focus in our sessions.

I am now driving the ball substantially further than ever before, and consistently hitting 290 to 300 yards. I am able to rotate further and use the improved strength of the key muscles to great effect.

Before I started working with Scott I had a severe shoulder injury; consistent lower back pain and my endurance were very poor. After 9 months, my shoulder has improved to the point where I no longer suffer and my golf swing is free and full. My back is now strong and pain-free, and my endurance levels are at an all-time peak.

Not only have the training sessions created fantastic results, but Scott's guidance on nutrition and lifestyle have helped me lose weight and improve sleeping patterns.

Kevin, **Property Developer**

"A life changing experience. One that has changed me"

Scott initially helped me with the support and guidance to get me through the initial stages of getting to know metabolic typing, following the six foundation principles and directing me in the right direction with exercise. There are particular methods used by C.H.E.K. professionals that have the most marvellous effect on body and mind. Scott guided me through the experience and showed me how to do this.

The therapeutic relationship that occurs between client and coach is one that comes to a place of understanding and empathy. This was certainly the situation with Scott and he has the ability to transcend that of the everyday personal trainer in a way that shows his high-level expertise and awareness as a Master C.H.E.K. Practitioner.

As a Metabolic Typing Advisor Scott took me through the process of assessing my needs in relation to healing my gut by arranging specimen to be sent, analysis of results and ordering the correct supplements to help with this. He also helped me analyse my food intolerances. This process takes time and I continue to have consultations with Scott in order that the process continues. I have adrenal fatigue and it takes time to recover from this. Depression has been a considerable issue with me -which goes hand in hand with the adrenal fatigue. Thanks to Scott's help in finding more deep-rooted reasons for my depression and by using methods of dealing with, it has been addressed in ways conventional medicine has never been able to. The improvement so far has been considerable and I feel the difference has made my life so much more enjoyable.

I was guided by Scott through different cleanses to detoxify my body. These cleanses have resulted in me feeling amazing and I realise that the commitment I have made through balancing my body chemistry with metabolic typing had to precede these cleanses – thanks to Scott's help. It was all a step change process and you very often have to be patient to get there. There is no quick fix, cookie- cutter approaches to how Scott works and you have to make the commitment to do it this way. This is far more effective than the tablet popping, behaviour controlling methods endorsed by conventional medicine.

Scott's Shamanic background has helped me deal with the blockages that occur within my body and mind – particularly due to past trauma. He has used methods that have helped considerably so far and I will continue to see Scott for the purpose of getting through the blockages that remain trapped in my body. I have every faith that Scott can help me with this.

My journey continues in the knowledge that Scott's methods will work and I will achieve the dreams in life that I wasn't by having and continuing to have a healthy, happy productive life.

Thank you Scott

Debbie Miller

1st August 2016

"Scott laid down the plan after reviewing my symptoms and within a few days I had my private stool sample sent out"

Have you got Parasites? Fungal infections? These are two very overlooked medical conditions that many doctors would pooh-pooh if you felt you had them (excuse the pun). I caught parasites for a variety of reasons and my GP did not believe me. The NHS stool tests are a waste of time as they only look for 4-6 parasites when there are 3500 recorded. I had nowhere to turn. Being a fan of the work of Holistic Health Expert Paul Chek, I searched for a C.H.E.K. certified master practitioner & found Scott. Scott is a master C.H.E.K. practitioner meaning unlike a nutritionist who is focused on nutrition, or a DR who is focused on the allopathic method, or a chiropractor etc focused on their skill he is well versed in all healing arts and views you as a holistic being. It turns out among having very low hydrochloric acid levels in my gut making me susceptible to parasites I had a lot of stress far more than was realised and ended up with adrenal fatigue too which destroyed my immune system. I had an initial consultation whereby Scott laid down the plan after reviewing my symptoms etc Within a few days I had my private stool sample sent out which is the world's best lab. I then started my lifestyle and diet review which is a few documents that need to be filled out over a week so Scott can really know where my health sticking points are. Moreover, we then did a metabolic type test which determines what foods your actually meant to eat for your genetic and geographical body type, quite incredible. Whilst I'm only two weeks in and about to start the metabolic type protocol to heal my issues such as gut and adrenals, and I am about to start the parasite cleanse shortly, Scott has saved me as I had nobody else to go to who had the experience or knowledge. Scott is also a Shaman and during sessions he has been helping me with belief, entitlement and my dreams. I can't be grateful enough and recommend him if you want to lose weight, get in shape, heal any illness or disease you name it Scott is your Master

Joel Ra

Scott started with a 4 hours body assessment in order to better comprehend why did my back problem start. that coupled with a 10 documents questions covering both past emotional events and diet/work environment questions. Scott has a tremendous good energy and is

24/7 dedicated to fixing your issues. Scott not only focus on strength and making you look better but also focus on balance/diet/wellbeing to achieve a truly healthy body from inside out. I highly recommend his service.

Lilia K

"A very good knowledge of how the body works"

Scott is super knowledgeable & passionate about the whole package. Exercise & Nutrition, all of it. He lives what he teaches and his enthusiasm runs deep. He is totally committed to your process. This is where you go when you are ready for a complete reboot. And it works!

Rina Malin

"I am finding Scott to be an excellent C.H.E.K. Master Practitioner

"I am finding Scott to be an excellent C.H.E.K master C.H.E.K. Business Mentoring, in the time I have been learning from Scott we have covered in depth the first stages of C.H.E.K system and also the 'day to day' aspects of a high-quality Personal Training/ HLC business.

Arron Page

Business Mentoring

I have been working with Scott for 6 months now. He is my coach, and my mentor in the C.H.E.K. Europe Academy, both of which he balances well. Before I met Scott I would have laughed at ideas (like every other misinformed, and close- minded person,) such as; Tai Chi, eating organic food, avoiding gluten, drinking half my body weight in warm water that was sourced from a natural spring, to name a few. His willingness to be persistent and teach me the value of such practices, has not only helped me grow to be more open-minded, he has helped me get rid of a leaky-gut that I have been carrying around (and trying and failing to fix a number of times with diet after diet,) for at least a decade. I would recommend Scott Bryant to any potential client, due to his extensive knowledge in diet, exercise, spirituality, and also the amount of love and care that he was lying dormant in his body, waiting to be projected onto you. You needn't look any further. Book a consultation, and get ready to grow into the energetic, healthy, radiant human being you never knew you could be...

Samuel Smith **C.H.E.K., Exercise coach**

Fast fat loss
Detox your body and mind
Banish back pain for life

Get your life together for post Brexit Britain 2019

WARNING

"The ideas contained in this book may change your life and help you realise your dreams . . . but only if you let them!"

CONTENTS

CONTENTS

This book is dedicated to my Dad and my sisters Tracey & Lisa.

To my long-time friends, teachers, coaches & gurus who have helped me see the big picture of life as well as giving me an open mind to see and feel more, enabling me to overcome obstacles in my life.

You helped me to keep my dreams alive.

Keep going and never give up on
your passions and dreams.

Acknowledgements

I would like to take this opportunity to thank all of the people who have helped and supported me during my 19-year career and with the writing of the book. My good friend Robin Allan, a sports therapy masseur, who has often kept me on an even keel and who introduced me to my fantastic ghost-writer and so got the book project underway. Doctors Roberto and Maurizio Viel, plastic surgeons to the stars, for their encouragement and for believing in me no matter what whacky courses I have taken. I'd like to thank Phil Loizides for being a wonderful friend; he is someone I've studied with and who has been very patient. A big thank you to Linda Mitchel, a good friend and a great client who has pushed me to write down my experiences and knowledge. I'd like to thank Arran Page, for helping write my blogs and for contributing opinions and ideas for this project. Thank you to Adam, a very nice guy, very hardworking and who inspired and pushed me to complete my level 3. Of course, I must express my deep gratitude to the Paul Chek Institute and Paul Chek in particular for helping me look at things in different ways, open my mind to new things, and understand that you can achieve anything in your life once you put your mind to it. I'd like to say an especially big thank you to all those clients I've worked with over the past 19 years who have let me help them with their fitness, health issues and lifestyles. And finally, I would like to thank the Universe for helping me live the life I do today and to keep living every day. Oh yes, I nearly forgot: thanks to my ghost-writer.

A Brief Biography

Scott's passion for health and fitness began at the age of just nine years old when his dad got him some chest expanders. Scott started reading fitness magazines back then when at home. At the age of 14 his teacher Oliver Caviglioli him how to lift weights and that really started something because he has been doing it ever since and for over 29 years now.

Scott had many different jobs before finding his true vocation. He had qualified as a chef by his early 20s, then went on to work as a doorman for a number of years in the pubs and clubs of the West End of London. But he grew tired of constantly being moved from place to place for the work and also of the constant stress and strain from dealing with all the violence and aggression to keep it from entering the venue.

When he reached 30 he realised he had to find something he loved and was really passionate about. That something had always been health and fitness and looking after himself, and so he decided to give it all up to become a personal fitness trainer with the YMCA London.

At first, Scott's dyslexia was an obstacle to his ambition because of the technical terms of anatomy and physiology that he had to learn. But one thing he had learned from weights was that to lift the heavier weights and get the bigger body you have to push yourself and not give up. And so he used this method in his studying, sometimes reading a book three or four times to get the knowledge in his head.

Quite soon after qualifying, Scott realised that although the YMCA fitness system was OK, it didn't get the results to work for some individuals with more complex issues. After a friend told him of the C.H.E.K. Institute at San Diego in California, Scott went out there in 2003 to meet the founder Paul Chek. C.H.E.K. was in fantastic shape, had a fantastic knowledge, and had brought out the CD set called You Are What You Eat.

After attending the C.H.E.K. seminar Scott took the CDs back home and studied them before putting the ideas into practice with his clients. He found they were losing weight, feeling better and understanding food at a much deeper level. He could see that the Institute was 10 to 15 years ahead of other systems, and so he began the 8-year programme to be a C.H.E.K. master practitioner.

While running his business he read and studied hard and eventually became the first of only two master C.H.E.K. practitioners new in the whole of the UK. Since qualifying, he has worked with everyone from TV and movie stars to golfers and bankers and has helped many clients achieve their aims.

Scott has had to overcome many obstacles on his journey to success and one of the greatest of these was dyslexia.

Qualifications and Achievements

Along with his 19 years of practical experience Scott has gained a number of formal and recognised qualifications.

At the C.H.E.K. Institute he gained the following qualifications:

Certified Master C.H.E.K. Practitioner
Shaman Practitioner
C.H.E.K. Practitioner level 1, 2, 3,4
C.H.E.K. Holistic Lifestyle Coach level 1, 2, 3
C.H.E.K. Golf Sports performance specialist
C.H.E.K. Exercise Coach
C.H.E.K. Europe Mentor 2 Years
Sports Massage Therapist
Chair Massage Therapist
Functional Diagnostic Nutritionist
Advanced Metabolic Typing Advisor Level 2
Y.M.C.A. Personal Trainer

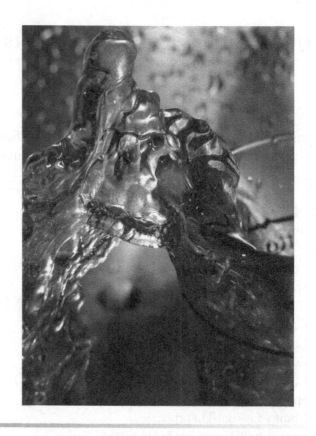

Positive Thought Positive Life

Detoxification: "Detoxify or Die!"

There are many tried and tested methods available out there on detoxification. Yes, you can diet, you can use steams, and you can use saunas. But what I like to do with my clients is to show them how to detoxify and cleanse the body over a period of one year. This is because conventional quick fixes simply do not work.

One of the best ways to detoxify the body is fasting, and various religions and cultural traditions have been using this method for centuries. Fasting is a way of relaxing the gut and forcing it to burn more body fat. It will cleanse both the organs and the mind and help to kill the parasites and fungi within the body. So you can see why I highly recommend it. And the good news is that most people will experience a euphoric effect after three days of fasting.

Intermittent fasting has been proven to help diabetes, insulin resistance, heart disease, and obesity. And in spiritual or religious terms, if you want to become more connected as some of us are through shamanistic practices, then fasting will help you become more spiritual.

I would suggest that intermittent fasting is the best way to start. For one day a week eat no food except bone broths and herbal teas with lots of water. When you have done this a few times you can move on to a three day fast. For this you may add soup to your fasting diet so that the body does not experience too much of a shock. During fasting you will be drinking your body weight in ounces of water, which will cleanse the kidneys and liver.

While you are fasting, you may add the practice of dry-skin brushing, which will cleanse the skin. Skin is actually the largest organ of the body. Incidentally, you may find that mild headaches are a side effect of dry-skin brushing but it is truly effective and really works. While fasting you may use steam or saunas, starting off with 5 to 10 minutes then eventually building up to 20-40 minutes to really remove the toxins from the system.

Now let's consider the bowel – this is the big one. You must cleanse the bowel before doing an intensive liver cleanse. If the bowel is not working properly and you are not doing three evacuations a day or producing 12 inches of faecal material a day, then technically speaking you are constipated. And so I would not recommend a liver cleanse under these conditions.

For liver cleanses, one method is to take a flannel, soak it in castor oil and put it in the oven until it gets quite warm. Then, place it in the region of the liver, wrap yourself in cling film, apply a heat pad, and hold it in place for 20 minutes. This will draw toxins out of the liver and purify it.

For cleansing the kidneys there are special additives and supplements but remember to use organic ones. There are also many parasite cleanses that can be obtained on-line for cleaning the gut. I take my clients through these processes nice and slowly to remove all the toxins from the body.

If you have toxins in the body you will be prone to skin problems (including cellulite), experience difficulty sleeping, and tend to have a poor memory. And so a detoxification programme is very important in conjunction with any exercise programme if you wish to attain peak health, fitness and wellness. We have only covered the basics here but will go much more deeply into things under instruction. You will appreciate the support and guidance, which will make sure you are getting it right and avoiding unnecessary injury.

So don't forget: detoxify or die. The choice is yours.

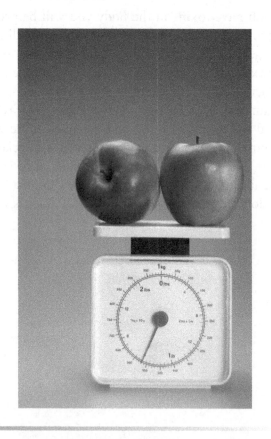

"Get out of your head and
get into your heart. Think less
and feel more" Osho

Diet and Lifestyle

Diet and lifestyle must come first in any health and fitness programme. If you don't change your diet and lifestyle, then don't expect your body to change even if you join an expensive gym.

The first thing I do with a client is to look at your diet using a system called the *metabolic typing diet*. In this system you are considered to be one of three types:

Protein Type: eating protein gives you more clarity and energy, and makes you feel great.

Carbohydrate Type: when you eat lots of vegetables and less meat you feel better and more focused.

Mixed Type: you need to eat equal amounts of protein and carbohydrates to increase your focus and energy and feel good.

The most important thing with any diet is obviously to eat good quality and healthy foods. I therefore highly recommend organic or biodynamic foods to my clients: frozen if you're on a tight budget but preferably fresh from the greengrocers.

7

How many people realise that they are unnecessarily frightened of fats? If we don't get enough fats inside our system our energy will be low, our skin will not look its best, our muscle mass won't increase, and our hormone levels may be low. Fat is really, really important. A book called *Cholesterol: The Myths* will help you understand that cholesterol is not something to fear. The body needs cholesterol to keep inflammation and swelling down. And fat gives us energy.

The good fats are:

Beef tallow
Lard
Butter
Olive Oil
Ghee

These are 5 different fats you can try with your meals to give you a good energy supply.

So with my clients I coach you on diet and lifestyle using metabolic diet typing and get you to balance the vegetables, proteins, carbohydrates and fats in your system to give you optimal energy. I also teach clients that water is key to the body's chemistry. 75 per cent of the planet is water and 75 percent of our bodies is water. The last sign of dehydration of the body is thirst. If you are thirsty then the body is robbing the water from your faeces in order to keep your body hydrated.

The next thing we need to look at with lifestyle is getting to bed on time. If you are not in bed by 10:30pm you will lose the advantage of the physiological and neurological repair of the body when the natural healing processes occur during the night. So you need to make sure that you switch off computers and phones before bed so that you can enter into deep sleep when you are in your bedroom.

Next with lifestyle comes exercise. I recommend to my clients at least 45 minutes of exercise four times a week to get the result you are looking for. You can do yoga, tai chi, weights, walking, anything in fact that you find fun and that you will always keep doing. But please note that some exercises do not give you the same benefit as others. If you're looking to develop muscle mass with tai chi, then it's not going to happen, nor will you get bigger and stronger with yoga. Similarly, if you're looking to lose weight but are only going walking, then unless you change the speed and the tempo of your pace you will not lose weight - even over a prolonged period of time. So I recommend my clients to do a combination of tai chi, yoga and strength training.

Remember that as you are aging you are losing muscle. Also your testosterone and other hormones are dropping. So weight or strength training for both males and females is very, very important. Muscles burn more calories than fat, so the more muscular you are, the leaner you will look and the younger you will feel. If you look at Olympic sprinters you will notice they have the best muscle mass and better toned bodies. They are doing strength and cardiovascular training in the one hit of the sprint.

There is now new research into H.I.T. training that demonstrates a simultaneous increase in speed, strength and cardiovascular conditioning from ten minute sessions. Personally I do not agree with this type of training. A preferable sequence is to warm up and stretch the body, followed by strength and conditioning exercises, and then cool down and stretch. This gives the best benefit.

As well as diet and exercise, rest is very important. I see many clients who are over training, overworking and under resting – this is why they are not getting the required results from their training programme.

So with your lifestyle programme, make sure you get to bed on time, eat according to your metabolic type, eat good fats, drink plenty of water, and spend time with friends doing what you enjoy most. And find a good C.H.E.K. practitioner to help you.

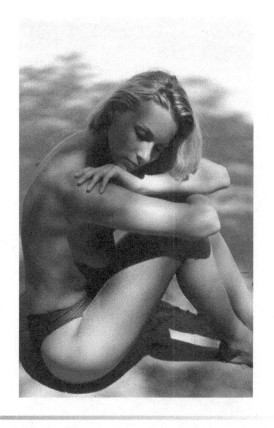

"Stay away from negative
people they have more problems
for every solution" Einstein

Corrective Exercise

Corrective exercise is an absolute must for anybody starting an exercise programme. It took me many years to discover this important fact. During all my 26 years of experience, corrective exercise was never mentioned! All instructors and colleagues ever spoke about was gaining muscle, getting bigger arms and legs, or becoming stronger, faster and fitter. I had picked up most of my training knowledge from friends, specialist magazines and from books like Arnold Schwarzenegger's *Encyclopaedia of Body Building*, a very insightful book with lots of heavy lifting exercises. But of course Schwarzenegger was doing tons of steroids in order to gain his muscle mass. I found these kinds of books didn't really work for me as I was training naturally, eating healthily and lifting weights hard.

Fortunately for me I was introduced to the C.H.E.K. method through a colleague at the gym where I was training. Since the C.H.E.K. Institute is based in California, the world centre of body building, I realised the method must have something. Paul Chek was using a corrective exercise programme along with a holistic diet and lifestyle system to get his world famous clients out of pain and back into sport. So this is when I became enlightened to the idea that corrective exercise has to be a number one priority in anybody's exercise programme.

While working out in all those gyms over the years I have made a habit of walking around and watching: I see people exercising without any training programme or any real direction, usually sitting at the machines with headphones on and reading newspapers. When I ask them why they have no exercise programme, they reply that it's all in their head. So then I ask: would you fix your car all in your head or would you read the manual, set out a plan and then decide whether to fix it or take it to a mechanic? If they answer sensibly then I ask them if they would like an exercise programme to correct their posture, help them look better, increase their energy and make them faster, fitter, stronger, and, most importantly, pain free. This is where corrective exercise comes into the training.

In the C.H.E.K. system Exercise Coach is one of four levels that we must reach before qualifying as a Master Practitioner. We learn to correct the body's alignment, switch on the core, and take the client through four distinct phases before we let them do the fun stuff. But the majority of gyms and trainers today take clients straight into speed and power, mistakenly believing they are doing their best for the client. But clients usually have faults that require correcting: faulty head-posture, inverted breathing, shoulder misalignment, anterior pelvic tilt, abdominal wall extension, or perhaps lower back, shoulder and knee pain.

And so in a corrective exercise programme everybody should follow the following sequence: flexibility, balance & stability, speed and power. As I have said, most people go straight into the last phases of speed and power: this is what Paul Chek observed during his 30 years of clinical experience. Going straight into speed and power is not the thing to do, and yet this is precisely what people do when they train in the park or join large fitness organisations. It is very wrong and very harmful to the body.

For the first stage of a fitness programme, FLEXIBILITY, the client must be assessed. I carry out 140 orthopaedic assessments of the body – so there is no guesswork involved. There are certain orthopaedic norms that need to be maintained in order to avoid injury. For example, if you have a tight hamstring or tight quadriceps, then this may be the root of your knee pain. If you have too much anterior pelvic tilt, postural tilt, or forward head posture, this may give you lower back pain. So you see, the body has to be individually assessed to find out what needs to be tightened, loosened or left alone.

The next part of a corrective exercise programme is STABILITY. Stability is about balance. A bad sense of balance will be setting you up for a future injury. For my corrective exercise system I use a lot of *Swiss Ball* work, which has been used by physios since 1953 to help people out of pain, although I tend to use it to strengthen individual muscles, stabilise the body and strengthen the core.

After the stability phase has been completed the client moves onto to the STRENGTH phase of exercise. Here the client develops strength and learns how to carry out *primal movement* patterns. The primal movement patterns consist of: squats, dead-lifts, pushes, pulls and rotations.

The next phase is SPEED. This is where we begin working faster now that the client's joints are stronger and more flexible and he or she has been taken out of pain. Clients seem to enjoy this phase when the tempo increases. Corrective exercise can be a bit boring for the client but once they start seeing improvements in their posture, in how they are moving, and become free from pain, then this really encourages them.

The last phase is POWER. Your power requirements will depend on your particular sport or pastime. Sprinters need extreme power; boxers need endurance as well as power; a yogi does not need physical power. Therefore every programme I design is tailored to an individual's particular needs. And so after the diet and lifestyle assessment there is a postural assessment lasting 5 hours in total: I am then fully equipped to write a fantastic programme for the individual. With a good corrective exercise programme I have been successful in removing shoulder, neck, knee and lower back pain.

But be warned: these corrective programmes can take time, and they depend upon how regularly the client is working with me. The minimum I will work with a client is twice a week because there is such a lot that I need to pass on. Additionally the client should train twice a week on their own. I have been using these corrective exercise programmes for about thirteen years and have found them to be hugely successful in getting clients stronger, faster and fitter: and they are very useful for removing pain in the shoulders, back and neck.

Unfortunately, when it comes to physiotherapy the therapists rarely understand exercise, and a physiological degree does not cover diet. In my clinical experience I have to find out where a client's pain is coming from. Could it their diet and lifestyle? Or perhaps a faulty or even non-existent corrective exercise programme? How about their posture? Or could it be connected with mental and emotional issues? I must assess you: if I am not assessing, then I am only guessing – which is what 85,000 trainers are doing in gyms all over the country. In my opinion, they are not doing a sufficiently in-depth study, and of course some may only be in it for the money.

I love my job and am passionate about getting the best for my clients. So corrective exercise is where we begin, taking you through the different phases in order to guarantee success in your sport or favoured activity. And I don't only train athletes, you know! I also train ordinary mums and dads, office workers, builders and anyone who's keen to exercise and get their body in shape.

So remember, if you do not have a corrective exercise programme then this maybe why you are not getting the outcome you really want. With a suitable programme, however, good results are guaranteed providing you pass through and complete the specific and necessary phases.

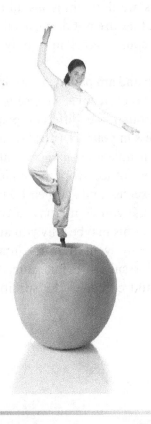

**Be somebody nobody
thought you can be.**

Holistic Body
Transformation for Women

Like many men, I've spent a lot of time admiring and loving women's bodies. But unlike a lot of men, I've also had to study and train women's bodies and help them lose fat, often when they themselves hold negative beliefs about their bodies and selves in general and therefore fear or even expect failure. And if women's husbands and partners instinctively dread that famous question: "Does my bum look big in this?", then please spare a thought for those of us who try and help women get the body they want.

The important thing for women to remember is that they have 20 percent more fat than males and their testosterone is lower. Therefore gaining strength and muscle can be difficult for women but it is nonetheless absolutely essential to gain muscle mass in order to replace fat mass. Since the female physique, nervous system and hormonal system are very sensitive, then when it comes to exercise women need to think outside the box.

Unfortunately the modern media preaches the idea that all women needs to do to keep in shape is a yoga class or a bit of running but I have found this to be completely untrue. When you run a marathon or even a shorter 10k run, you convert your body into a *calorific*

burner, not a *fat* burner. And if you look closely at the
average marathon runner you will notice that they are
fatter than either a sprinter, weightlifter or cross-fit
exerciser. I've seen women cross-fit training with
explosive lifts and strength conditioning to get optimum
and awesome results. But the drawback with cross-fit
training is that women can damage their hormonal
system and muscle-skeletal system quite easily because,
as I have said, their bodies and systems are much
more sensitive than men's bodies, which have higher
testosterone and growth hormone levels and a greater
proportion of muscle mass.

If we go back 10,000 years to hunter gatherer
societies, we find that men were the hunters and women
were the gatherers. It is important to understand that
we cannot simply override thousands of years of
evolution. And yet here in the modern age we see many
women gravitating towards yoga. But unfortunately the
women that enjoy yoga tend to be the ones who are
hyper-mobile and 98 percent will have lower back pain.
So if you are really looking for a holistic approach and
you really want to get your body in shape and keep it in
shape as you age, here are my suggestions.

Firstly, consult a professional to find out what your
metabolic type is, or perhaps try out the Atkins diet.
If eating too much protein gives you a headache and
makes you feel crap, and you gain more body fat, then
you are a carbohydrate type: so you need to eat more
carbohydrates. But if you try the metabolic typing diet
and you eat like a protein type, which is more meat than
carbs on the plate, then your body changes. Or if you do
the Atkins diet and your body changes dramatically and
your energy levels increase, and you are broad in the

shoulders with a skinny waist, then these are the tell-tale signs of a protein type.

Many women exercise extremely hard in the gym but do not get the result they are looking for because they have not addressed their diet. If the human body is more complex than a car engine, then why would you not bother to have a proper exercise program? Unfortunately such questions don't always go down too well and lead to complaints to the management. So really, if you are a cardio junky and want to keep your cardio going but are worrying from the previous paragraph that you will gain fat mass, then this is what you should do: one minute on, one minute off. That is, train hard for one minute and lightly for the second minute, so that you give your body time to recover. You only need 15 to 20 minutes of this to get optimum results.

Scientific research has found that during *hit training* the body only needs to train hard for 10 or 15 minutes to get optimum results. This should mean that I become unemployed very quickly. But no, because we still all need to stretch and mobilise, and we all need to go through certain conditioning to keep our body injury free (see section on Corrective Exercise).

So if you truly want a specific body shape, and to lose fat and gain muscle mass, you must remember that no woman, I repeat, no woman, can gain huge amounts of muscle mass like a female body builder does – unless of course they use synthetic drugs. No woman can gain huge muscle amounts of mass without taking testosterone supplements or other synthetic drugs. I've heard this so many times that it makes me upset to hear women say: "I don't want to get all big and muscly on your programme." So I have to gently point out that they've been reading the wrong magazines and have not educated themselves properly. They may find this a bit insulting but I'm just being truthful.

When it comes to getting back your holistic body, yes, I recommend yoga: as long as you're not hyper mobile or in pain. But yoga is not the only answer: you need to do specific weight training to burn calories, break down muscle mass, or break down muscle and rebuild it slowly over time. If you look at superstars like Madonna, J-Lo, and some of the big athletes, you will notice that as they age they retain their body mass, which keeps them looking young. There's an article about Madonna on my website where you can read how she combined yoga, running, weight lifting and dancing to keep her body in shape. She has truly done that: she is 60 and still looks amazing.

The other thing that women have to take into account is that as you age your oestrogen level will drop but your testosterone will increase, which is why a lot of women when they reach 50 have to shave because of these higher levels of testosterone. But if you train regularly, then that testosterone can be converted into muscle and strength, and you can have a wonderful body in your 50s, 60s and even in your 70s – Madonna is proving this.

So here are my four top tips:

One, women must weight train to maintain muscle mass and bone mass. Women often gravitate towards alcoholic drinks with coco cola, lemonade or other fizzy drinks, which affect PH levels and take calcium out of the bones, which can cause arthritis as you age. So weight training to keep muscle mass and keep lean is a must for any women.

Two, get your hormones checked. Find out if your hormones are at the level they should be or if you have any problems that may be preventing you from gaining muscle and strength.

Three: never miss a meal. Every time a woman misses a meal her body fat will increase because we are designed to be able to survive famines. Every time you miss a meal your body will multiply its fat cells and you will get bigger rather than leaner. So eating regularly and according to your metabolic type is essential for any female.

Four: make sure you get plenty of rest. Older ladies may suffer from night sweats, insomnia, and may therefore find excuses for missing sessions with their trainer. So it's important to get adequate sleep, which is usually 6 to 8 hours, in order to feel fully recovered from exercise. The hormone check will find out if your adrenal glands are functioning properly so that when you are lifting weights and doing your cardiovascular interval training you will be able to gain lean muscle over all of the body.

I find it is adequate for women to train regularly four times a week to enhance their bodies to the degree they desire: twice yoga, twice weights, or once yoga, three times weights. The old fallacy was that we need to combine cardiovascular training with weight training, but the latest scientific findings show that while weight training we will tone up the cardiovascular system, strength and hormones all at the same time. So if you don't have time for cardio exercise you should do strength and conditioning in the gym to get that great looking body and to look and feel youthful.

I am a great believer in fish oils and supplements to keep brain chemistry balanced. A good multivitamin will help you feel good. And never miss meals. But if you are someone who wants to lose vast amounts of body fat very quickly, then I highly recommend fasting: I've been using this method on myself and my clients for years now and find it to be absolutely essential for getting the body back in shape, balancing hormones, or attacking the onset of diabetes or obesity. So if you are obese and want to get back into shape, or you have diabetes, breathing problems, or hormonal imbalances, you will find that fasting will allow you to balance everything. But fasting can be very hard to do, so perhaps you may need a coach to show you what to do and take you through the different stages of fasting.

So ladies, I hope you have enjoyed this section of the book.

"I am willing to believe in my ability to heal." Scott Bryan

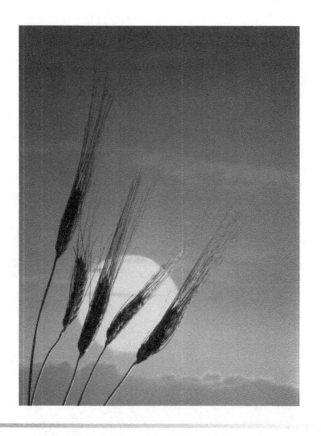

"I am willing to believe in my
ability to heal" Scott Bryant

Shamanism

Technically speaking, the word shaman is restricted to the ritual and healing specialists functioning in the clans or tribes living on the Russian steppes. More generally the word is used to refer to the healing practitioners of archaic cultures which go by many names according to the particular time and place where they occur: medicine men, witches, witchdoctors, druids, call them what you will. Scholars believe shamanism is the oldest religion in the world, but I don't really see it as a religion: I don't have to read a bible, I don't have to stop doing the things I enjoy, and there are no rules and regulations. All you need to be a shaman is an open mind and a willingness connect with others and give compassion and love.

Why do I use shamanic techniques with my clients? Well, I have found over the years that clients often have personal blockages that act as barriers to their success, and these blocks are not just about food, lifestyle or exercise. People also have family problems or mental and emotional issues that prevent them from adhering to a training programme. In some cases clients have been suffering long-term pain which no one has previously been able to remove. I really enjoy this aspect of my work as here we do not allow intellect to get in the way of healing. Instead, we just let things come in naturally and then respond to them.

While studying on my Master's Practitioner course I worked with Paul Chek, who is himself a shaman and applied his training to my particular issues. First of all we worked on the voice and its overtones. Next, I lay down while he used rattles and incense to *smudge* my body. He also held stones over different parts of my body and clashed them together, using the sound to diagnose and heal. I felt totally different after the session and was told to expect more changes in the following days when I returned to England.

During level 4 of the course Paul had introduced us to Native American drumming. I got a bit carried away and started using my voice as well, singing overtones and working through the chakras. After this, Paul nicknamed me the sound Buddha as my voice was, and always has been, strong. When I got back to England I made up my mind to research shamanism at a deeper level, and contacted a South American shaman called Alberto Villoldo who had founded *The Four Winds Society*. Being a former doctor and an anthropologist, he understood health at a very deep level. This skilful and well educated man often found that people in his clinical practice would not heal or get better because of the medical drugs they were on. He had been looking at the brain and the effect upon it from drugs. He came to the conclusion that the drugs were not working to heal the diseases.

Being an anthropologist, he began studying and working with shamans all over the world but mainly in Peru. A Peruvian shaman explained that we need to have more healers on the planet and so they have decided to release knowledge of their system called *The Nine Rites*, which has been passed down through shamanic families for generations. These rites allow the shamanic practitioner to power up the chakras and strengthen the body from the inside out. The techniques can be passed on to anybody who is ready for them.

In the system I use I map out the whole body to find out where the problem or illness is coming from. To find the root cause of the problem I use the data and paperwork that the client and I have gathered together while working on the holistic lifestyle aspect of the course. This normally takes 10 days. Next, I dowse the chakras to find out which ones are not functioning in the right way. After the dowsing, I enter the spiritual healing space that the traditional shamans work in and seek their help to balance and realign the body. I use various implements to carry out the work, such as: rattles, stones, crystals, sage and other herbs, etc.

I have used this system successfully on many clients. One client, for example, had blockages over money. After applying shamanic techniques on him in his office he was able to get out of the red and back into the black and resolve his financial issues. Another client was closed off in relation to her own needs. After using the techniques she opened up more and learnt the value of rest and of not overworking.

In Western society you need a certificate for everything these days before people will believe in you. That's why I decided to study with Alberto Villoldo in London and learn the Nine Rites. I will always use these techniques if the client is open and ready for them but will not force these things onto people in any way. I try to meet the client where they are and consider what they are ready for. I help them understand that these are healing techniques that we may use and which work well.

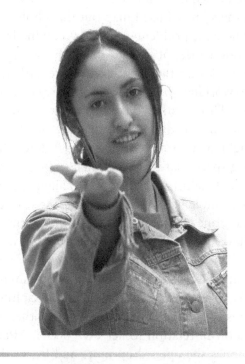

"Create a vision of who you want to be and live into that picture as if it were already true"
Arnold Schwarzenegger

How To Stay Focused And
Not Give Up On Your Dreams

Here are my five top tips to avoid self-sabotage.

Tip Number One: YOU MUST HAVE A DREAM.

What I mean by a dream is: where would you like to be five or ten years from now? Do you want to look back on your life with joy and happiness, knowing that you've achieved something each year and always kept moving forwards? The dream can be anything from being fit, healthy and lean, to being the best golfer in the world or even becoming a multimillionaire.

All you need to do is to learn to focus and open up your mind. Spend ten minutes a day, every day, thinking only about your dream. But do not think about how hard it is to achieve it or worry where the money might come from or some other detail. I've found in my own personal experience that by staying focused on the dream, the money and circumstances just appear. But when they appear you must see them and act on them straight away!

My dream to become a master C.H.E.K. practitioner took 12 long years of staying focused but not all goals need take so long. I achieved my goal and so I know you can achieve your goals using the same system, whether your goal is weight loss, fitness, sports performance, or anything else. This system has been used by Steve Jobs, Richard Branson, Tony Robbins, and many world famous movie stars and pop stars.

If you listen carefully to what these people say on the telly and the radio, and in their music and films, you'll notice that they always talk about the dream and staying focused on it. So I feel this is a number one priority if you want to achieve something in your life. You have to see and feel the dream, stay focused on it, and never let the naysayers hold you back.

Tip number two: HAVE GOALS.

If you do not have goals you are doomed to failure. You can have big or small goals. I've found using small goals to achieve the bigger ones is a real winner. Saying your goals in your mind, out loud, or writing them down, helps your subconscious mind to download what you want in your life. Writing down 90 day goals can help you achieve anything.

Goals have to be realistic for you to make them become a reality and it is how you say the goals that is really important. So if you say "I will be a millionaire," the Universe notices the "will be" part and so may not give you what you want because it remains in the future. But if instead you say: "I *am* a millionaire, I *am* financially free, I *have* lost weight, I *am* fit and healthy," then with repetition your subconscious mind will download it, act on it, and make it a reality. I learnt about goal achieving through the audio programmes of two self-made millionaires called Bob Proctor and Brian Tracy.

Tip Number 3: VISION.

You need to visualise the big dream and the goal becoming reality. Spend 15 minutes a day doing deep breathing and letting your mind wander without judging what comes in. For example, if a vision comes in of a massive house, big cars and a swimming pool, be careful not to say in your mind: "this isn't going to happen, it isn't real." Embrace the vision, let it happen and become reality.

I found that by being in the moment, really feeling the vision and repeating it over the days, months and years, then the vision becomes a reality. I found that day dreaming is one of my big secrets. When I daydream about new clients and keeping myself fit so that I can help others, then it always works. So put 15 minutes of visualising into your daily schedule to become more successful and achieve your big dream.

Tip Number 4: BELIEF: SELF BELIEF CAN ACHIEVE

A book called *The Mind Gym* is used by elite athletes. They visualise and believe they have already won the trophy. Similarly, the business man visualises and believes he has landed the deal. I believe you must ask the Universe, God, Spirit or whatever you believe in, to help you achieve your big dream. When we open our minds to the Universe, the Spirit, or even fairies perhaps, because it really doesn't matter what we call it, then our dream is more likely to happen.

There have been times over the years when I had no money or clients and things were very, very tough. But I kept believing within myself that things would change and get better, and that this was just a test. It has always worked and I have always come bouncing back. And

I have also found that the tougher the time has been, then the easier it is next time around. So believing in yourself is so, so important for getting your body back into shape, for thinking at a different level and living in a better way.

As well as believing in yourself it is important to have people around you who believe in you and your dream: people that are going to help you focus and go forward in your life. You don't want negative people and naysayers around you that may stop you from achieving your dreams, goals and ambitions. So believe in yourself today and you will change your life forever.

Tip Number 5: DO NOT GIVE UP.

Throughout my career I have found that when training in the gym or studying at home and on courses that things have often been very difficult for me because I am dyslexic. But it is only as tough as you let it be. So by never giving up you will be able to achieve anything. I left school with no qualifications. I am now 48 and have over 15 qualifications to my name. I have been reading, learning and studying, and training in gyms all over the world. I've been knocking down walls of negative beliefs, thought patterns and attitudes about myself for many years now. I have realised one important fact: never give up.

So whether you want to get that six-pack, lower your golf handicap, get out of pain, lose weight or get fit, then as long as you do not give up then you will eventually succeed. If you have had a problem in the past but have always given up before solving it, then it is fantastic that you have found my book. So find my website, get on the phone, give me a call, and we can work on your dreams, goals and visions, and I will personally make sure that you never give up on yourself. That's what I'm here for.

I always ask my clients: "What level of change are you ready for on a range from 1 to 10?" If you are a one, then you are definitely someone who needs more help than I can give. But if you are at a level of seven to ten, then you are definitely someone I can help. So have a good think about that: are you ready for change? Are you ready to knock down the walls of self-sabotage and change your life for ever? I am a caring and compassionate guy and love what I do with a deep passion. If you'd like to start on your life goal today, then give me a call.

Scott Bryant

Appendix

The Transcendency of Drumming

Scott Bryant CP4

In Fulfilment Of
C.H.E.K INSTITUTE MASTER THESIS

Dreaming The Drum

Drums are a dream arisen,
Weaving the tapestry of life.
Drums bear seekers of vision,
Embracing the rainbow of light.

...Cherokee

"Sacred drumming generates harmonic resonance - a synchronization of two or more tones. It is the weaving of harmonic overtones that repairs the sacred tapestry of life. Fundamental harmonics of vibrational frequency waves structure our physical reality as well as alternate realities. Everything in the universe vibrates at a specific resonant frequency, which is an integral multiple of the voice of the creator, the fundamental frequency, underlying all manifestation. A coherent cycle of frequencies is an octave and it is octaves of waveforms that structure matter. The structure of an atom can hold only eight electrons (an octave). The shell is complete and another expansion must occur in order to create a new shell or harmonic zone, which again fills up to a maximum of eight electrons.

More and more complex structures are created through a repetition of octaves of waveforms. The universe is composed of a symphony of waveforms with the harmonics played on a vast range of octaves. All aspects of matter and reality can, therefore, be manipulated, altered or transmitted resonantly as harmonic overtones. Using the drum one can work it so that it sings and hums. Synchronize your intent with these frequency overtones. Resonate with the divine octave of ecstasy"

I consider myself to be a modern, yet spiritual man. I feel the connection between the earth and myself through my Chakras and have not felt closer to my spirit self and the earth as when I drum. The vibrations I feel from the drum are, to my clients, and me so much more tangible than the spiritual vibrations of my imagination. I can actually feel and recognise shifts in my Chakra and increase my own proprioception through the act of drumming and meditating (allowing us to ask and answer internal questions) by using the drum.

The human body (as with every other living organism) has a frequency. Different densities within the body (influenced by tension, posture, body shape etc.) will limit how resonance can travel through the Chakras. The body, from my experience, needs to be aligned and unblocked in order to be at its healthiest and most efficient. I have found and will show how drumming allows this transformation through aligning the Chakras and focussing the mind.

The importance of the drum is closely tied to its tremendous importance as an early social tool. The drum would call together tribes during times of need, and for moments of celebration. The drum announced war and carried other important messages over distances greater than the voice could carry. With this in mind, it is easy to see why the drum would become thought of as an 'earthly voice' for the Spirit (in fact, in reading the histories of everyone from the Bedouins to the Israelites, that's what the drum became, and certainly this is its function in the neo-pagan movement today.)

To understand the drum in its modern forms, we need to see it in its historical settings. Let us begin with the ancient Greeks, where we find an interesting religious practice. The priests and priestesses here were the only ones allowed to beat out an iambic-pentameter on the drum or any other sacred musical instrument. This particular beat was thought to be very powerful in how it affects people, and it was considered dangerous and inappropriate for anyone else to use it. Nonetheless, the Greek and Roman followers of Dionysus and Cybele used frame drums regularly as part of worship.

In Shamanism, the drum is regarded as an incredibly important tool. It is relatively safe to say that if you seek out a Shaman, you will also find a drum. Shamans from Siberia to Africa and beyond use this implement to transport the Shaman into the spirit realm. The sound of a drum focuses the practitioner and bridges the gap between the mundane and magical world. For example, Eskimo Shamans use drums for ecstatic rites (often in hunting rituals or to inspire visions), but they also have a more relaxed approach for simple contemplation where they actually sleep with the drum.

Lapland has a similar tradition where the Shamans used a drum covered with runes and seemed to fall into a trance while sounding it. When the Shamans awoke, they could tell about their travels and any information they retrieved in the other realms. On a rather sad note, early Christians saw the Laplanders' drums as tools of Satan, each of which had a demon within that cast a spell when beaten. This led to the burning of many beautiful family treasures in the 17th Century.

During ecstasy perhaps one of the most important functions of a shaman's drum occurs - that of soul travel into other realms to retrieve important information for a person, the land, or a whole tribe. Typically during their travels, shamans seek out familiar spirits, power animals, and guides for assistance. To accomplish this communion and achieve a deep trance, the shaman drums and sings, allowing the drumming to shift and change with every spirit he or she encounters in the voyage. In this manner those listening nearby indirectly experience the shaman's inner landscape. Throughout the whole experience the drumbeats carrying the shaman express what's happening to him or her and also leads the shaman back to normal awareness at the end of the ritual.

In many ancient settings drums were considered "female" and the drumstick "male" so that the two working together symbolised the most powerful of creative forces. Among the Urok Indians it's customary to give away your first drum to someone else. Receiving it is an honour. In Navajo writings, the drum is the Great Spirit's favourite instrument, and that is why humans have a heartbeat. When used in ritual context, Tabi Drums (Qatar) are believed to have the power to heal. Another tribal belief is that dabbing the head of a drum with blood increases the power of the drum (and also binds it to you). In some regions of the West Indies people believe that a drum will not sound until special invocations are spoken over it (here the drum is the voice of god).

The drum also symbolised the family unit. So when they met and beat the drum, it synchronised the family into a coherent and emotionally connected 'whole'. Allowing the individuals to feel a closer connection to each member of the family.

The symbiotic genesis of dance and drum is incontrovertible. Before stringed or wind instruments (excluding the human voice) were first created, the beating of time for the purpose of dance was made on wood and even using crudely fashioned stretched animal hides. Changing a rhythm affects heart rates and could alter the participants physiology even when there was no scientific understanding of this process. Dancing and drumming stimulate all the senses in a wordless way - the heart and soul have rhythm. The Celts have a saying. "In the fiddler's house everyone dances" I think the same could be said for drummers and dancers too - Aloma (aka the Pixie).

The myths of dance are as rich to the eyes and ears as the dance itself. We begin our exploration with the sun dancer myth from the Mayan tradition:

"One day a man discovered a beautiful array of clothing just sitting unattended. The clothes shone with vibrant golds, yellow, reds and oranges. He was so enamoured with the clothing that he couldn't resist trying it on, only to discover himself under a spell. He began to dance and dance around the forest and dance and dance through the glade. At last he came to the edge of a cliff, but he did not fall. Instead the dance led him upward to the sky, where he (in all his splendour) becomes the Sun, and he continues to dance to this day."

Meanwhile, in Japan we discover the Kabuki theatre, the roots of which begin in Shinto tradition and myths of Amaterasu, the Sun goddess. According to the stories, the first dances of this type re-enact the moment Zhen Uzume (the goddess of merriment), seeing that Earth needed warmth, determined to coax Amaterasu out of her cave.

She did so by dancing wildly and making all the other gods and goddesses laugh and applaud. When Amaterasu heard the noise, she moved outward only to see a reflection of herself in a mirror, which gave the gods and goddesses enough time to move the door and let the Sun back into the world.

The song "Lord of the Dance" goes, "Dance, dance wherever you may be, for I am the Lord of the Dance said he." While there are several divine beings to whom this song could be dedicated, Shiva might fit the lyric best. This god is forever dancing the 'ananda tandavam', the dance of bliss, symbolising the five divine acts of grace, concealment, dissolution, sustenance, and creation. So important is dance to the worship of this god that his temples throughout India include dance halls. India is certainly not alone in such customs.

Scholars believe that dance was one of the earliest languages of humankind, and dancing as a spiritual methodology goes back to Neolithic times (at least 9.000 BCE). It is safe to say that dance was present at all the important moments of human life. From Hungarian courtship, to Polynesian friendship rituals, Polish wedding dances, African work rhythms, Guatemalan vegetation leaping, Chinese healing movements, Mexican rain rituals, Eskimo hunting rites, Tibetan animal mimes, and Borneo war dances, there are very few eras or cultures on this planet that have not been touched by the spirit of the Dance.

In their earliest forms, dances represented the transformation of space and time and the creative force of the universe. Round dances, in particular, mirrored cosmic and seasonal cycles to insure life's continuance, patterning themselves after the movement of the Sun, Moon and other celestial bodies. For example, Etruscan dance was specifically designed to keep the stars on course. Circular dancing also reflected the round of seasons, to which, out of necessity, early people were far more attuned. By comparison, chain dancing connected people to each other, particularly men to women for fertility and humans to the earth as our source of sustenance. And thread or ribbon dances speak of fate and uncovering the mysteries (by finding our way in and out of life's maze).

If one wants to experience the sacred dance there are guidelines that one can follow to help immerse oneself into the spirit of it and aid the journey into an uninhibited focus.

Sacred Dancing Guidelines

- Warm up physically, emotionally and spiritually to the task ahead (doing those all important motivational checks)
- Move into the circle slowly, treating it reverently. Consider entering from the south, so that you're moving toward the fire in harmony with your space in the wheel.
- Take the time to become aware of other dancers and overall feeling/flavour of the movement
- Integrate yourself into the circle, pace yourself against the fire, the drum and the other dancers.

- Release yourself to the tempo, and if you wish, add other rhythmic accompaniments (clapping, chanting, song, etc.).
- As you go, don't overlook your body's needs. When you begin to get thirsty, get water from the fire tender. When you're tired, rest a while.
- Listen to the leadings of Spirit, then translate that energy into your movements.

The Therapeutic Effects of Drumming

Drumming as a therapeutic technique has already been used for thousands of years to create and maintain physical, mental, and spiritual health. Current research is now verifying the therapeutic effects of ancient rhythm techniques. Recent research reviews indicate that drumming accelerates physical healing, boosts the immune system and produces feelings of well-being, a release of emotional trauma, and reintegration of self. Other studies have demonstrated the calming, focusing, and healing effects of drumming on Alzheimer's patients, autistic children, emotionally disturbed teens, recovering addicts, trauma patients, and prison and homeless populations. Study results demonstrate that drumming is a valuable treatment for stress, fatigue, anxiety, hypertension, asthma, chronic pain, arthritis, mental illness, migraines, cancer, multiple sclerosis, Parkinson's disease, stroke, paralysis, emotional disorders, and a wide range of physical disabilities.

Research studies mentioned in this thesis exemplify that drumming: reduces tension, anxiety, and stress. Drumming induces deep relaxation, lowers blood pressure, and reduces stress. Stress, according to my C.H.E.K training as well as my clinical work and current medical research, contributes to nearly all disease and is a primary cause of such life-threatening illnesses as heart attacks, strokes, and immune system breakdowns.

Drum therapy is an ancient approach that uses rhythm to promote healing and self-expression. Current research is now verifying these therapeutic effects of ancient rhythm techniques. The gentle pulsating rhythms (binaural beat) of our brain is accessed in modern therapies by the introduction of synchronization tapes. These act in a similar fashion to the brains natural rhythms, yet because the frequencies are computer generated, they are precise, consistent and can be targeted to induce highly specific and desired brain states. Much like tuning a radio to get a particular station, our brain synchronization tapes can induce a variety of brain states. Effecting Alertness, Concentration, Focus & Cognition Relaxation, Visualization, & Creativity Intuition, Memory, Meditation Vivid Visual Imagery, Deep Sleep, Detached Awareness.

There are frequencies/rhythms, which when dominant in the brain, correlate with a specific state of mind. There are generally 4 groupings of brain waves.

1. Beta waves range between 13-40 HZ. The beta state is associated with peak concentration, heightened alertness and visual acuity. Nobel Prize Winner, Sir Francis Crick and other scientists believe that the

40HZ beta frequency used on many Brain Sync tapes may be key to the act of cognition.

2. Alpha waves range between 7-12 HZ. This is a place of deep relaxation, but not quite meditation. In Alpha, we begin to access the wealth of creativity that lies just below our conscious awareness – it is the gateway, the entry point that leads into deeper states of consciousness. Alpha is also the home of the window frequency known as the Schumann Resonance, which is the resonant frequency of the earth's electromagnetic field.

3. Theta waves range between 4-7 HZ. Theta is one of the more elusive and extraordinary realms we can explore. It is also known as the twilight state which we normally only experience fleetingly as we rise up out of the depths of delta upon waking or drifting off to sleep. In theta we are in a waking dream, vivid imagery flashes before the mind's eye and we are receptive to information beyond our normal conscious awareness. During the Theta state many find they are capable of comprehending advanced concepts and relationships that become incomprehensible when returning to Alpha or Beta states. Theta has also been identified as the gateway to learning and memory. Theta meditation increases creativity, enhances learning, reduces stress and awakens intuition and other extrasensory perception skills. When the brain is in Theta it appears to balance sodium/potassium ratios, which are responsible for the transport of chemicals through brain cell membranes. This appears to play a role in rejuvenating the fatigued brain.

4. Delta waves range between 0-4 HZ. Delta is associated with deep sleep. In addition, certain frequencies in the delta range trigger the release of Growth Hormone beneficial for healing and regeneration. This is why sleep, deep restorative sleep, is so essential to the healing process.

Drumming produces deeper self-awareness by inducing synchronous brain activity. Research has demonstrated that the physical transmission of rhythmic energy to the brain synchronizes the two cerebral hemispheres. When the logical left hemisphere and the intuitive right hemisphere begin to pulsate in harmony, the inner guidance of intuitive knowing can then flow unimpeded into conscious awareness. The ability to access unconscious information through symbols and imagery facilitates psychological integration and a reintegration of self.

Drumming also synchronizes the frontal and lower areas of the brain, integrating nonverbal information from lower brain structures into the frontal cortex, producing according to Winkelman: "feelings of insight, understanding, integration, certainty, conviction, and truth, which surpass ordinary understandings and tend to persist long after the experience, often providing foundational insights for religious and cultural traditions."

Another recent study found that a program of group drumming helped reduce stress and employee turnover in the long-term care industry and might help other high-stress occupations as well.

1. Helps control chronic pain. Chronic pain has a progressively draining effect on the quality of life. Researchers suggest that drumming serves as a distraction from pain and grief. Moreover, drumming promotes the production of endorphins and endogenous opiates, the body's own morphine-like painkillers, and can thereby help in the control of pain.

2. Boosts the immune system. A recent medical research study indicates that drumming circles boost the immune system. Led by renowned cancer expert Barry Bittman, MD, the study demonstrates that group drumming actually increases cancer-killing cells, which help the body combat cancer as well as other viruses, including AIDS. According to Dr. Bittman, "Group drumming tunes our biology, orchestrates our immunity, and enables healing to begin."

3. Produces deeper self-awareness by inducing synchronous brain activity. Research has demonstrated that the physical transmission of rhythmic energy to the brain synchronizes the two cerebral hemispheres. When the logical left hemisphere and the intuitive right hemisphere begin to pulsate in harmony, the inner guidance of intuitive knowing can then flow unimpeded into conscious awareness. The ability to access unconscious information through symbols and imagery facilitates psychological integration and a reintegration of self. Drumming also synchronizes the frontal and lower areas of the brain, integrating nonverbal information from lower brain structures

into the frontal cortex, producing "feelings of insight, understanding, integration, certainty, conviction, and truth, which surpass ordinary understandings and tend to persist long after the experience, often providing foundational insights for religious and cultural traditions."

4. Accesses the entire brain. The reason rhythm is such a powerful tool is that it permeates the entire brain. Vision for example is in one part of the brain, speech another, but drumming accesses the whole brain. The sound of drumming generates dynamic neuronal connections in all parts of the brain even where there is significant damage or impairment such as in Attention Deficit Disorder (ADD). According to Michael Thaut, director of Colorado State University's Center for Biomedical Research in Music, "Rhythmic cues can help retrain the brain after a stroke or other neurological impairment, as with Parkinson's patients..." The more connections that can be made within the brain, the more integrated our experiences become.

5. Induces natural altered states of consciousness. Rhythmic drumming induces altered states, which have a wide range of therapeutic applications. A recent study by Barry Quinn, Ph.D. demonstrates that even a brief drumming session can double alpha brain wave activities, dramatically reducing stress. The brain changes from Beta waves (focused concentration and activity) to Alpha waves (calm and relaxed), producing feelings of euphoria and well-being. Alpha activity is associated with

meditation, shamanic trance, and integrative modes of consciousness. This ease of induction contrasts significantly with the long periods of isolation and practice required by most meditative disciplines before inducing significant effects. Rhythmic stimulation is a simple yet effective technique for affecting states of mind.

6. Creates a sense of connectedness with self and others. In a society in which traditional family and community-based systems of support have become increasingly fragmented, drumming circles provide a sense of connectedness with others and interpersonal support. A drum circle provides an opportunity to connect with your own spirit at a deeper level and also to connect with a group of other like-minded people. Group drumming alleviates self-centeredness, isolation, and alienation. Music educator Ed Mikenas finds that drumming provides "an authentic experience of unity and physiological synchronicity. If we put people together who are out of sync with themselves (i.e., diseased, addicted) and help them experience the phenomenon of entrainment, it is possible for them to feel with and through others what it is like to be synchronous in a state of preverbal connectedness."

7. Helps us to experience being in resonance with the natural rhythms of life. Rhythm and resonance order the natural world. Dissonance and disharmony arise only when we limit our capacity to resonate totally and completely with the rhythms of life. The origin of the word rhythm is Greek meaning "to flow."

We can learn "to flow" with the rhythms of life by simply learning to feel the beat, pulse, or groove while drumming. It is a way of bringing the essential self into accord with the flow of a dynamic, interrelated universe, helping us feel connected rather than isolated and estranged.

8. Provides a secular approach to accessing a higher power. Shamanic drumming directly supports the introduction of spiritual factors found significant in the healing process. Drumming and Shamanic activities produce a sense of connectedness and community, integrating body, mind and spirit. According to a recent study, "Shamanic activities bring people efficiently and directly into immediate encounters with spiritual forces, focusing the client on the whole body and integrating healing at physical and spiritual levels. This process allows them to connect with the power of the universe, to externalize their own knowledge, and to internalize their answers; it also enhances their sense of empowerment and responsibility. These experiences are healing, bringing the restorative powers of nature to clinical settings."

9. Releases negative feelings, blockages, and emotional trauma. Drumming can help people express and address emotional issues. Unexpressed feelings and emotions can form energy blockages. The physical stimulation of drumming removes blockages and produces emotional release. Sound vibrations resonate through every cell in the body, stimulating the release of negative cellular memories. "Drumming

emphasizes self-expression, teaches how to rebuild emotional health, and addresses issues of violence and conflict through expression and integration of emotions," says Music educator Ed Mikenas. Drumming can also address the needs of addicted populations by helping them learn to deal with their emotions in a therapeutic way without the use of drugs.

10. Places one in the present moment (Rudolph Steiner). Drumming helps alleviate stress that is created from hanging on to the past or worrying about the future. When one plays a drum, one is placed squarely in the here and now. One of the paradoxes of rhythm is that it has both the capacity to move your awareness out of your body into realms beyond time and space, and to ground you firmly in the present moment.

11. Provides a medium for individual self-realization. Drumming helps reconnect us to our core, enhancing our sense of empowerment and stimulating our creative expression. "The advantage of participating in a drumming group is that you develop an auditory feedback loop within yourself and among group members-a channel for self-expression and positive feedback-that is pre-verbal, emotion-based, and sound-mediated." Each person in a drum circle expresses themselves through his or her drum and listening to the other drums at the same time. "Everyone is speaking, everyone is heard, and each person's sound is an essential part of the whole." Each person can drum out their feelings without

saying a word, without having to reveal their issues. Group drumming complements traditional talk therapy methods. It provides a means of exploring and developing the inner self. It serves as a vehicle for personal transformation, consciousness expansion, and community building. The primitive drumming circle is emerging as a significant therapeutic tool in the modern technological age.

Drumming also has powerful physiological effects. Most obviously, sustained drumming increases the heart rate and blood flow, resulting in the "high" common to any aerobic exercise. There are also more subtle effects. In an article in the drum newsletter "Reach Into the Pulse", Layne Redmond discusses the effect of drumming on the synchronization of the brain's two hemispheres. The process of drumming engages both the linear, rational left-brain (in the learning of polyrhythmic parts and the analysis of how rhythms fit together) and the creative, intuitive right brain (in the entrainment of rhythm in the body and the appreciation of the music). The two brain hemispheres often emanate different wave frequencies; drumming, like deep meditation, brings them into synchronization, which is experienced as an opening of consciousness. Redmond writes, "Synchronized brain wave activity with very high amplitude alpha waves can create feelings of euphoria with a sense of expanded mental powers and flowing creativity... This may be the neurophysiological basis of what are called 'higher states of consciousness'."

Tom Bickford of Spiritcraft Drums conveys a related idea when I ask him why he drums. A drum builder, healer, and shaman, Tom says that shamanic journey drumming directly links humans with the vibration of the Earth by slowing the brain waves to around 8 cycles per second, the same frequency as the planet. "Drumming heals the human energy field, exactly like the laying on of hands," he says. "It energizes and clears the chakras. If your intention is for healing to happen when drumming, it will. Immersing oneself in the energy field of shamanic journey drumming is tremendously healing to all aspects of human beingness, physical, emotional, mental and spiritual." The bottom line, he says, is that drumming "makes you feel good. It opens you up to the heartbeat of Mother Earth. Why do I drum? So I can hang out with Mom."

Although shamanic journey drumming is different from the polyrhythmic drumming that has its origins in African cultures, the energetic impact on humans is the same: it induces an altered state (sometimes called "trance", sometimes "ecstasy") that opens the way for healing or transformation. This altered state is the realm of the shaman, the one who seeks the guidance of spirits to effect change. When people are drawn to the drum they intuitively feel its potential to change them, though they do not always consciously understand it.

Jimi Two-Feathers, co-founder of Earth Drum Council, believes that drumming and dancing around the fire is the original, primal consciousness altering experience for human beings. "The nightclub of modern times is an attempt to duplicate that primal feeling," he says, "but there is no substitute. Humans walk, breathe, have a heartbeat -- we are basically rhythmic beings, and drumming taps into that. When you create that magical space around the fire where everyone has the same information, the same understanding of how the circle of energy works, then people become more at one with each other, more whole. The junk falls away, people become more honest on a soul level, and can unfold and fly. The drum circle has elements of entertaining and being entertained, but it's also the original church. In that space people can experience real transformation."

The healing and transformation created by drumming can be quite striking. Bob Bloom describes himself as "a drummer guy who does it because of the people it leads me to meet." After years of studying and then teaching African drumming, Bob is now working with the Rhythm for Life Foundation, focusing on bringing drumming to people with illness and disabilities, the elderly, and the very young. Bob gets intense pleasure from seeing the effect that playing with drums and percussion instruments has on people. His voice is animated as he describes giving an egg shaker to a man with cerebral palsy, who began to play it instantly and giggle with delight. In cases like this, the healing is not abstract or ethereal, but immediately observable.

Music therapy

Music therapy, when combined with standard treatment – is effective in helping people with depression, according to a Finnish study. Researchers from the University of Jyväskylä believe that making music can help people express their emotions and reflect their inner experiences. Their findings are published in the August issue of the British Journal of Psychiatry.

The research team, led by Professor Jaakko Erkkilä and Professor Christian Gold, recruited 79 people aged between 18 and 50 years old who had been diagnosed with depression. 33 of the participants were offered 20 music therapy sessions, in addition to their usual treatment for depression. In Finland, standard treatment for depression includes medication (antidepressants), 5-6 individual psychotherapy sessions and psychiatric counselling. The other 46 participants just received standard treatment and acted as the control group.

The one-on-one music therapy sessions each lasted 60 minutes and took place twice a week. Trained music therapists helped each participant to improvise music using percussion instruments and drums. On average, each participant attended 18 music therapy sessions. 29 (88%) attended at least 15 sessions. The participants in both groups were followed up at 3 months and 6 months and assessed for symptoms of depression and anxiety.

The researchers found that, after 3 months, the participants who received music therapy showed greater improvement than those who received standard care only. They had significantly fewer symptoms of depression and anxiety and scored better on general functioning. Although improvements remained after 6 months, the difference between the groups was no longer statistically significant.

Professor Gold said: "Our trial has shown that music therapy, when added to standard care including medication, psychotherapy and counselling, helps people to improve their levels of depression and anxiety. Music therapy has specific qualities that allow people to express themselves and interact in a non-verbal way – even in situations when they cannot find the words to describe their inner experiences.

Professor Erkkilä said: "We found that people often expressed their inner pressure and feelings by drumming or with the tones produced with a mallet instrument. Some people described their playing experience as cathartic. Our findings now need to be repeated with a larger sample of people, and further research is needed to assess the cost-effectiveness of such therapy."

UK experts have welcomed the research. Writing in an editorial in the same issue of the British Journal of Psychiatry, Dr Mike Crawford, Reader in Mental Health Services Research in the Centre for Mental Health, Imperial College London, said: "This is a high-quality randomised trial of music therapy specifically for depression, and the results suggest that it can improve the mood and general functioning of people with depression. Music making is social, pleasurable and meaningful. It has been argued that music making engages people in ways that words may simply not be able to."

BBC News has reported, "Music therapy can be used to improve treatment of depression, at least in the short term". This story was based on a trial in which people being treated for depression with standard therapy were also given 20 one-hour music therapy sessions. During the sessions they could play a mallet instrument, a percussion instrument or an acoustic, West African djembe drum. After three months, patients receiving music therapy had a significantly greater improvement in their symptoms than those who had only received standard therapy. However, assessments made a further three months after the therapy finished showed that these differences were no longer statistically significant.

Depression is usually treated with medication and psychiatric counselling. Previous studies have found that music therapy is a promising additional treatment for depression. This was a well-designed trial that demonstrated the potential benefits of music therapy. However, it was a small trial with only 79 participants over a three-month treatment period. Longer, larger trials are required to confirm this finding and to determine the best length of treatment.

Where did the story come from?

Researchers from Finland and Norway carried out the study. Funding was provided by the NEST (New and Emerging Science and Technology) programme of the European Commission, and the Centres of Excellence in research at the Academy of Finland. The study was published in the peer-reviewed journal The British Journal of Psychiatry. This story was well reported by The BBC and The Daily Telegraph. The Independent covered the story accurately, but its headline suggested that music therapy is a cure, which is not the case. Although the study found an improvement in symptoms with music therapy, the difference was not significant after treatment finished.

What kind of research was this?

This randomised controlled trial aimed to compare the efficacy of combined music therapy and standard care with standard care alone in adults with depression. This is the most appropriate type of study design to answer this sort of question.

What did the research involve?

The study looked at 79 participants with diagnosed depression aged between 18 and 50. Participants were included irrespective of what medication they were taking and were allowed to continue with their medication during the study. They were randomised to receive either standard care with music therapy (20 sessions in total, with two sessions every week) or standard care alone.

Active music therapy involved individuals being invited to play either a mallet instrument, a percussion instrument or an acoustic djembe drum. During each hour-long session, the therapist and the patient both had identical instrumentation. The therapists were all professionally trained in music therapy according to Finnish training standards.

Standard care consisted of short-term psychotherapy (five or six individual sessions) conducted by nurses specially trained in depression, medication and psychiatric counselling.

Clinical measures of depression, anxiety, general functioning, quality of life and alexithymia (the ability to understand, process or describe emotions) were measured at the start of the trial. They were then measured at the end of the music therapy sessions (three months after treatment began) and again three months after the treatment had finished by a clinical expert who had not been told which of the participants had been given which treatment.

The main scale used to measure depression was the Montgomery–Asberg Depression Rating Scale, which is a 10-item questionnaire with scores ranging from 0 to 60. Other scales were used to assess anxiety and general functioning.

What were the basic results?

Of the 79 participants, 33 were allocated to receive music therapy with standard care. A total of 12 participants dropped out from the trial before the three-month follow-up and another three before the final follow-up, three months after treatment finished. The dropout rate was higher in the control group (receiving standard care) than in the music therapy group.

Individuals in the music therapy group attended an average of 18 out of 20 sessions, which is a high attendance rate.

After three months, scores from the three scales showed that those receiving music therapy plus standard care showed significantly greater improvement than those receiving standard care alone.

- Scores of depression symptoms (ranging from 0-60) improved on average by 4.65 more with the music therapy than standard care alone (95% confidence interval [CI] 0.59 to 8.70).

- Scores of anxiety symptoms improved on average by 1.82 more with music therapy than standard care alone (95% CI 0.09 to 3.55).
- Scores of general functioning were improved on average by 4.58 more with music therapy than standard care alone (95% CI 8.93 to 0.24).

When the authors defined a "response" as a 50% or greater reduction in the depression symptom score, they found 45% (15/33) of people responded in the music therapy group compared to 22% (10/46) in the control group: a difference of almost 24%. This was statistically significant (odds ratio 2.96, 95% CI 1.01 to 9.02). The improvements observed were clinically relevant. The researchers calculated that, for every four people to whom music therapy is offered, one will have a "response".

However, when measurements of depression, anxiety and general functioning were taken three months after the treatment had finished, the differences between the scores were no longer statistically significant.

How did the researchers interpret the results?

The researchers concluded that, "individual music therapy combined with standard care is effective for depression among working-age people with depression". They determined that these findings, along with those of previous research, indicate that music therapy is a valuable addition to established treatment practices.

Conclusion

Depression is commonly treated with medication and psychiatric counselling. Previous studies have found that music therapy is a promising additional treatment for depression. This randomised controlled trial demonstrated that people receiving active music therapy in addition to standard care had a significantly greater improvement in their symptoms than those receiving standard care alone after three months of treatment. There are some points that are worth noting:

- This was still a small trial in only 79 participants, of whom 33 received music therapy. Larger trials will be needed to confirm the results.
- The treatment period was only three months. Longer trials are required to confirm the best length of treatment, as in this trial there were no statistical improvements three months after treatment had ceased.
- When the authors defined a response as a 50% or greater reduction in the depression symptom score, they found 45% (15/33) of people responded in the music therapy group compared to 22% (10/46) in the control group, a difference of almost 24%. If this is confirmed in further studies, it suggests that music therapy could provide important benefits.

This well-conducted small trial has shown that music therapy may be of some benefit as an additional treatment for depression, in combination with standard therapies. However, the benefit from this relatively short trial period only remained statistically significant while the people continued to have these therapy sessions. In the context of the other trials listed in a Cochrane review, the results suggest that a larger trial of longer-term music therapy is needed.

Extract from presentation on relevant research by Melinda Maxfield, Ph.D.

"The purpose of the research was to determine whether various drumming patterns would be associated with different brain wave activity, as measured by cortical EEG, and to determine if the subjective experience of percussion in general, and rhythmic drumming, in particular, would elicit images or sensations with a common theme.

Twelve participants were divided into three groups and monitored for EEG frequency response to three separate drumming tapes. These tapes included: Shamanic Drumming, at approximately 4 to 4 1/2 beats per second; I Ching Drumming, at approximately 3 to 4 beats per second; and Free Drumming, which incorporates no sustained rhythmic pattern. Four cortical sites, bilateral parieto-temporal and parieto-central areas, were monitored for each participant during three sessions. At the conclusion of the sessions, each participant prepared a brief written account and was given a tape-recorded interview of his or her subjective experience. These subjective experiences were then categorized according to recurring themes and consensual topics.

This research supports the theories that suggest that the use of the drum by indigenous cultures in ritual and ceremony has specific neurophysiological effects and the ability to elicit temporary changes in brain wave activity, and thereby facilitates imagery and possible entry into an ASC (altered state of consciousness), especially the SSC (shamanic state of consciousness).

Drumming in general, and rhythmic drumming, in particular, often induces imagery that is ceremonial and ritualistic in content and is an effective tool for entering into a non-ordinary or altered state of consciousness (ASC) even when it is extracted from cultural ritual, ceremony, and intent. The drumming also elicits subjective experiences and images with common themes. These include: loss of time continuum; movement sensations, including pressure on or expansion of various parts of the body and body image distortion, "energy waves," and sensations of flying, spiralling, dancing, running, etc.; feelings of being energized, relaxed, sharp and clear, hot, cold, and in physical, mental, and/or emotional discomfort; emotions, ranging from reverie to rage; vivid images of natives, animals, people, and landscapes; and non-ordinary or altered states of consciousness (ASC), whereby one is conscious of the fact that there has been a qualitative shift in mental functioning., including the shamanic state of consciousness (SSC) journeys, out-of-body experiences (OBEs), and visitations.

A pattern that incorporates approximately 4 to 4 1/2 beats per second is the most inducing for theta gain. (Theta frequency is usually associated with drowsy, near-unconscious states, such as the threshold period just before waking or sleeping. This frequency has also been connected to states of "reverie" and hypnogogic or dream-like images.)

The pattern of the drumbeat as it relates to beats per second can be correlated with resulting temporary changes in brain wave frequency (cycles per second) and/or subjective experience, provided the drumming pattern is sustained for at least 13-15 minutes."

Drumming away Dis-Ease

In the beginning of all life there was sound and rhythm... Every atom, particle, and molecule is in constant vibration, and therefore has a frequency. The whole universe, including all living creatures is in a state of vibration or in other words made of sound. Sound is the first of our senses to develop and the last that leaves us when we die. In the womb we are constantly bathed in our mother's body sounds like her heartbeat, respiration, digestion, voice, to list only a few. Every organ, cell, bone, tissue and liquid of the body and also the electromagnetic fields which surround the body (aura), has a healthy vibratory frequency. If we are not resonating with some part of ourselves, or our surroundings, we become dissonant and therefore unhealthy and "dis-ease" can manifest. This century, the Western world has rediscovered and scientifically proven what ancient cultures and tribes already knew for thousands of years, sounds and music can heal us.

In Africa, the continent of human origin and roots of all music, the drum was the primary form of communication. Beside that the drums and their rhythms were used for socialization, entertainment, dancing and healing the planet and the people who dwell upon her. Many mythologies speak about the drum as the shaman's most important tool in healing rituals to induce a state of trance, which is the primary key to eliminate any state of Dis-Ease.

Psychologists have long studied rhythm's effects on our psyches. Robert Assiogoli, Ph. D., who in 1908 founded Psychosynthesis, a holistic discipline in psychology, he notes that ancient people used the drum and rattle to increase the effectiveness of herbs and also used the instruments alone to promote healing. Furthermore, the drum is the most accessible musical instrument. No other instrument gets people as immediately involved in a successful music making experience as the drum. Through the drum, all kinds of goals can be addressed, be they physical, cognitive or emotional. A variety of problems – including depression, stress, high blood pressure, addictions, asthma, migraines, Alzheimer's disease, cancer, multiple sclerosis, Parkinson's disease, stroke, paralysis, autism, Down Syndrome, William's Syndrome and a range of physical disabilities – are currently treated with music and especially drumming.

Sound and rhythm interacts with our mind, body and soul on at least 4 levels:

1. Psycho-acoustic effect on the brain. The brain can change from Beta waves (hard concentration and focused activity) to Alpha waves (calm and relaxed) to Theta (deep relaxation and visualization). During this process the logical left hemisphere of the brain is gradually switched off and the intuitive and creative right hemisphere is activated.

    Drumming increases our Alpha brainwaves, those brainwaves associated with feelings of well-being and euphoria. Dr. Barry Quinn, a licensed clinical psychologist found out that especially his hypervigilant (highly stressed) patients benefited from drumming, as Alpha waves doubled after only 30 minutes, immediately after the first drumming session.

The reason that rhythm and music is such a powerful tool is because it accesses the brain globally. Vision for instance is in one part of the brain, speech another, but music uses the whole brain.

2. Physical effect on our body. Research revealed and confirmed that music therapy affects the production and release of neurotransmitters and neurohormones like melatonin, epinephrine, serotonin, and prolactin into the bloodstream...such increased levels may have contributed to patients relaxed and calm mood.

Follow up research from other sources showed that drumming, especially in groups, alters neuroendocrine and immunologic measurements in the participants.

Cortisol level, normally increased under stress, was down on all trials and blood pressure levels are reduced while drumming. Natural killer cells, responsible for attacking viruses, etc., showed an increased activity after drumming sessions. Researchers suggest that drumming promotes the production of endorphins, the body's own painkillers, and can thereby also help in the control of pain.

3. Psychological and spiritual effects. Sound vibrations resonate through every cell in your body, allowing

the energy centres to realign and to release negative cellular memories.

Drums and their rhythms can align and balance mental, emotional and spiritual energy bodies, balance chakras and enable emotional blockages and imbalances to be shifted.

This also has a profound effect on our consciousness, raising our vibrational level and enabling us to access spiritual dimensions.

Through hitting the drum, unhealthy and toxic emotions can be released. The drum, then, becomes a tool of alchemy, altering that which is negative into something positive through an action as simple as a drum slap.

As many healers have taught since the time of Pythagoras, when we move with the flow of life, we reduce stress and help our minds and bodies function, as they are intended to. When we go against that flow, life becomes difficult and we suffer, first emotionally and later physically. Learning to feel the rhythm, pulse or groove while drumming can help us to actually experience that flow in ourselves and in others. Ultimately, to flow with the pulse, to be in a groove activates our own natural desire for health, which is the most important step to achieving it.

The drum provides us with an ancient form of communication, one that does not rely on the articulation of words, but one that uses a much more basic language, our emotions expressed through sound. When people communicate verbally, they are limited to one-way communication (one person speaking and others listening), and there is great room for miscommunication and misinterpretation.

When a group of people are drumming together, everyone is speaking through his or her drum and listening to the drums at the same time. Everyone is speaking, everyone is heard, and each person's sound is an essential part of the whole. The drum seems to have the capacity to unite all individuals who choose to experience it together and creates an experience of wholeness and community. Despite race, religion, colour, creed, background, or ideology, all are joined together through this ancient instrument's calling.

The drum and its rhythms unlock some of the most positive qualities we have as human beings – the need to connect with others, the expression of our creative selves, the exhilaration of joy and play and the potential to heal.

Naming and Decorating the Drum

One should decorate the drum to personalise it in order to make it an extension of one's self (this can include leaving the drum as is or buying a pre-decorated drum that 'speaks to you'). As for decorations, some drums love bells and whistles, while others don't wish to be adorned. Unlike the mundane world, plainness does not equate to less power here. It's a sign of respect for the Drum Spirit's wishes. In fact, sometimes the lack of adornment only makes the drum more beautiful. A spiritual drummer does not go around dressing up a drum like a doll to please the ego. Instead, if we adorn them, adornment has meaning.'

'Decorating one's drum has a long and respectable history. For example, the shamans in the South Pacific use pod rattles and lizard skins to enhance sound. Aztecs carved their drums to look like animal spirits (on whom the shaman called for aid). North American drumheads were often painted with images of rainbows, clouds, sunshine, stars and other symbols of the natural world. West African drummers put metal rattles (looking like bent paddles with rings) on their djembe before going into battle, not only to create a unique sound and appearance but also to protect themselves from spears and arrows.

Types of decorations

Here are just a few examples of possible decorative touches that can help one connect spiritually with the drumming:

1. Elemental Touches on the head (like a string of shells in the West, a feather in the East, earthen beads North and incense South.)
2. Special symbols or relief carvings patterned into the wood.
3. A vibrating chord or stick over the hollow as both decoration and a way of providing alternative percussion. (percussive effects)
4. Bells or jingles added to the sides
5. Henna paintings on the head
6. Permanent paintings on the head (warning: this can change the tone of your drum) or the body of the drum.

7. Specialised coverings that either temper the sound of the drum or protect it in storage
8. Braided or otherwise specially made strings around the drumhead or for use as carrying harnesses.

Drum Healing Case Histories

1. Sharon, 50 years of age. *Myalgic Encephalomyelitis*

In my initial assessment I found that she had no energy, was stressed out and had no money. Her father had died and she was now looking after her mother in a full time capacity. I used a Tap, Tone, Tune assessment to look at her first Chakra energy.

She presented with financial insecurity, tribal ties through family and an inability to achieve her goals indicating a weak 1st Chakra.

The 2nd Chakra was strong, indicating strong sexual energy but low fluid balance.

The 3rd Chakra indicated that she was weak in her power and self-will because her diaphragm had shut down; she found it hard to achieve her dreams.

The 4th Chakra was closed down because of a split with a lover after 12 years, as the 4th Chakra is all about giving and receiving love. She also found it hard to internalise compliments regarding love.

The 5th Chakra showed that she is a strong communicator but verbalising her self-will is weak.

The 6th Chakra was strong in universal intelligence and strong in creating and developing new ideas. However, it was weak on emotional intelligence.

The 7th Chakra was transcendent, indicating a strong bond with her higher self, but her dogmatic belief system seemed to be blocking her.

I also found she had weakness with her breathing, winging scapulae, hyper-extended abdominal wall, fungus on the tongue (indicating the likelihood of fungal and or parasite infection).

Due to her financial difficulties she could not afford to let me use the full C.H.E.K system to heal her, so I chose to use drumming as an effective and affordable alternative, especially as she seemed receptive to the technique and had even received sound healing before from another practitioner (although not a C.H.E.K Practitioner).

I started by getting her to lie on the Massage table, then to take 10 deep diaphragmatic breaths (as best she could) and just relax. I felt her energy using my intuition and discerned the areas of blockage that needed attention. I found that she was quite Yang with her energy (leading from her current situations). So I put coloured silk, representing each individual Chakra, on the energy centres and then placed Chakra crystals on top of those. I cleansed the crystals the night before using Smudging and a Tibetan bowl. I began the healing session by using a Native American Rattle up and down her body 7 times per Chakra. Then I went around the body 7 times in a clockwise direction with the same Rattle.

My intuition then led me to move on to the **Drum**, I played it with a slow, quiet rhythm progressing upwards to a fast, loud rhythm following my client's responses and her increasing acceptance to the rhythmic changes. The next intuitive step I made was to add my vocal resonance to the drumbeat in order to balance her energy more efficiently. Then I started to transmit healing love and other positive energies. My next course of action was to Smudge, starting at her feet and blowing the smoke over the length of her body. After this I allowed her to settle as I said a 10-minute prayer.

Once I finished the prayer the next intuitive step was to use the 7th Chakra tuning fork over her body in order to reaffirm and rebalance her energy field. Once I had restarted the resonant part of the treatment I decided to continue it with my voice (using overtoning) whilst all the time still transmitting healing love energy. After this I filled a Tibetan Bowl with water and played it for approximately 5 minutes. As I finished playing the bowl I felt as though we were approaching the natural conclusion to the session, and so chose to carefully bring her back to full consciousness by counting back from ten and slowly getting her to open her eyes. She then slowly sat up where I then placed a healing crystal on top of her head and placed the top Chakra tuning fork on top of that. The end of the session came as the tuning fork's resonance had fully dissipated. At which point I provided the client with water to make sure that she was fully hydrated.

CLIENT Feedback:

"Scott, this was a unique experience. You are truly gifted. I'm not sure what you've done but I feel absolutely amazing... Rebalanced... Reenergised. I need to definitely come back again for more." (Which she has!) Since the first treatment she has been able to support her life with nutritional supplements, which I recommended, and she has made more positive strides in her life (including a more successful love life).

2. Tom, 28 years of age. *High Stress and a Left Brain Dominance.*

I have known Tom for 5 years and we got together after I finished my C.H.E.K level 4. He was very stressed due to some exams he was about to sit and could not 'get out of his own head'. I took this opportunity to take him to the park and introduce him to the Drum. As he was a friend I decided to use the drumming session to also allow myself to enjoy the Drum.

We started off with Chi exercises to warm us up and make us more receptive to the experience (also so we could leave the drum in the sun to warm it up in order to allow the skin to stretch).

After 20 mins of these exercises we then picked up the drums. Tom was a tad apprehensive and self-conscious to begin with. But once he began to listen to the beat, at my instruction, he began to relax more and let himself get absorbed into the session. I, at this point, was beginning to feel euphoric and totally relaxed as did he (we even joked that it felt similar to smoking dope). The session was drawn to a close in a slightly unnatural way due to the time restraints on Tom. So, in order not to end the session abruptly, I chose to end using a Tai Chi Ruler exercise. The purpose of this was to teach him about his breath, due to the fact that his stress and the beginning of the release of his sympathetic system needed help. The Tai Chi Ruler exercise seemed like the most appropriate exercise to do at the time.

CLIENT Feedback:

"The drumming made me feel really relaxed, far less stressed over my exam… I feel more able to face and hopefully ace my exam"

(which he did)

My observations of self after participating in the session were that I felt very chilled and relaxed whereupon I moved to sit under a beautiful tree where I drew a Mandala. It was so nice to not only experience the drum with another person but to see the power of the drum in others. It opened me up and combined our spirits for that moment.

4. Yeshovardhan, 30 years of age. *Poor Familial bonding. Weak power and self-will.*

Yesho has been a client of mine for a while and has previously presented with back, neck, shoulder, gut, knee issues and "stinking thinking" about himself. I have successfully used the C.H.E.K program to rebalance and reenergise Yesho of these issues. However his familial issue with his father and his left-brain dominance (lack of faith in himself or belief in a greater being) was still prevalent.

So we began with Chi breathing for 20 mins. whilst the drums heated up in the sun. So, as we had 2 drums of differing frequencies we switched between drums, rhythms and dancing positions. I then got Yesho to lie down on the grass while I drummed and overtoned on his weaker Chakras. He then lay there for 5 minutes absorbing the sun's Chi whilst I sent loving healing energy his way.

He then stood up slowly, at which point we over-toned together making our way through all his 7 Chakras. We visualised the Chakra colours as we progressed through each point opening him up and grounding him firmly using the overtones and stamping. This led us to the natural conclusion of the session. We ended by hugging and sharing our energy and positivity.

CLIENT Feedback:
"It was the best session we've ever had, why didn't we do this before? It was fantastic"

To which I replied that he wasn't receptive enough beforehand and may have been scared off. I believe the reason why this session was so successful, was because of his receptive state at the time. Since this session, he now sings in the shower every day and hugs his father far more often. He even says that he can now see love all around him.

In conclusion, based on my own experiences, and on the research, I feel strongly that in order to find mental and physical balance the most efficient and all-encompassing technique, which has been with us as a species for Millennia, is Drumming. The effects of drumming are manifold, soothing the spirit and connecting us to the world that surrounds us. Enabling us to see and experience the bigger picture with a positive outlook.

"Ten individuals, sharing a common goal, would therefore have the power of one hundred individuals. Even a small group of people of one mind, one purpose, and fully attuned through the drums, can transform the world and manifest what is needed to benefit all beings"
–Michael Drake

During my education of the drum and integration into my business as a senior C.H.E.K Practitioner, I have been inspired to use it more often as a vital tool in healing and it has opened my mind to the healing properties of resonance and vibrations. It has opened my eyes to the intricate relationship between the body's energy flow and the flow of these vibrations throughout the body (as a healing tool and as a diagnostic one also). This has led me to a realisation that vibrations from other instruments (such as the voice and even resonant phonations from other sources) could have a similar affect, which I am very much looking forward to exploring, and incorporating into my existing practice.

Ah Ho, Great Spirit!

References

1. Ash, Steven, & Ash, Renate. (2004). *Sacred Drumming*. Sterling.
2. Bittman, M.D., Barry, Bruhn, Karl T., Stevens, Christine, MSW, MT-BC, Westengard, James, and Umbach, Paul O., MA. "Recreational Music-Making, A Cost-Effective Group Interdisciplinary Strategy for Reducing Burnout and Improving Mood States in Long-Term Care Workers." *Advances in Mind-Body Medicine*. Fall/Winter 2003, Vol. 19, No. 3-4,
3. Bittman, Barry, M.D. "Composite Effects of Group Drumming...," *Alternative Therapies in Health and Medicine*. January 2001, Vol 7, No. 1:38-47.
4. Bittmann, Simonton. Simonton Cancer Center. CA. USA. (2001).
5. Cattan, Rogelio MD, Et.al. Music therapy increases serum melatonin levels in patients with Alzheimer's disease. *Alternative Therapies in Health and Medicine*. November 1999, Vol. 5:6.
6. Diamond, John. (1999). *The Way of the Pulse - Drumming with Spirit*. Enhancement Books, Bloomingdale, IL.
7. Drake, Michael. (2007). *The Tao of Drumming*. Talking Drum Publications.
8. Drake, Michael. (1991). *A Guide To Sacred Drumming*. Talking Drum Publications.

9. Erkkilä J, Punkanen M, Fachner J, Ala-Ruona E, Pöntiö I, Tervaniemi M, Vanhala M and Gold C. "Individual music therapy for depression: Randomised controlled trial." *British Journal of Psychiatry*, April 7, 2011, 199:132-139.

10. Friedman, Robert L. (2000). *The Healing Power of the Drum*. White Cliffs, Reno, NV.

11. Hart, Mickey. (1991). *Planet Drum – A Celebration of Percussion and Rhythm*. Harper Collins, New York. NY.

12. Maratos A, Crawford MJ and Procter S. "Music therapy for depression: it seems to work, but how?" *British Journal of Psychiatry*, April 7, 2011, 199: 92-93.

13. Maxfield, M. PhD. (1990). *Effects* of *rhythmic drumming* on *EEG* and *subjective experiences*. Unpublished PhD Dissertation, Institute of. Transpersonal Psychology, Menlo Park, CA.

14. Mikenas, Edward. "Drums, Not Drugs." *Percussive Notes*. April 1999:62-63.

15. Telesco, P. & Waterhawk, D. (2012). *Sacred Beat: From the Heart of the Drum*. Circle Red Wheel.

16. Winkelman, Michael. "Complementary Therapy for Addiction: Drumming Out Drugs." *American Journal of Public Health*. Apr 2003, Vol. 93(4) 647-651.

17. Winkelman, Michael. (2000). *Shamanism: The Neural Ecology of Consciousness and Healing*. Westport, Conn: Bergin & Garvey.

About the Author

Scott has been working out in gyms all over the world for over 34 years.

He is a Level 4 certified Master C.H.E.K. Practitioner and has been personally training pop and movie stars, sportsmen and women, golfers, mums, dads and kids too. With his 19 years' experience, he has also been coaching and mentoring other personal trainers and C.H.E.K. practitioners to be the best they can be.

Scott has read over 600 books on health, healing, diet & lifestyle, fitness coaching & sports performance. He has taken over 42 courses and workshops on the aforementioned topics as well as being a shamanic practitioner.

Scott was featured in the Guardian newspaper, Women's Magazine & golf online. He also featured in *The Viels' Beauty Bible*, where he contributed to health and wellbeing.

Currently, Scott is working on his new book to be released in 2020 on exercise, dyslexia and the business mind.

Are you ready to make your dream a reality?

Please write below details of your ONE primary goal:

_____

_____

_____

_____

_____

1. <u>Questionnaire</u>

    1. Have you tried many doctors, coaches and personal trainers? But you are still not achieving your goals?
    2. Would like to sleep more and have more energy?
    3. Are you in pain and need help?

If have answered yes to 2 or more of these questions then call us on 07841144878
or email scttbrynt@aol.com

Or live chat on web site

https://activebryantsystems.com/

A free gift for you!

Get the body and fitness you want with your free online fitness programme.

You can use it anywhere in the world to get fit and it will be personalised for your body.

To find out more, live chat with us on site or use the free code 666 666 to get your free online fitness programme when you call or email us. This offer is limited to the first 100 people.

Call Scott on phone number 07841144878,
Email scttbryn@aol.com
Or go to https://activebryantsystems.com/

Thank you for reading my book.